Leptin Diet For Women

Best Leptin Diet Recipes To Reset Your
Leptin Levels

By Kathy hunt

Introduction

Welcome to this beginners guide on the leptin resistance diet and an introduction to some amazing recipes that you can whip up in no time. Inside this 45 minute read you will definitely find some golden tips and tricks on how to deal with leptin resistance and will bring you to a whole new overall better healthy lifestyle.

Each section of this book has been designed step by step to take you by the hand through each chapter so you have a true understanding of taking your health and body to where exactly you want it to be.

Let's get started!

Kathy Hunt

Introduction

Chapter 1 – Introduction to leptin and leptin resistance

Chapter 2 – Leptin resistance diet (what to eat what to reduce)

Chapter 3 – Breakfast recipes

Raspberry vanilla oatmeal

Tomato borscht

Kale salad

Roasted beet and goat cheese salad

Chapter 4 – Lunch Recipes

Chicken Chili

Crab salad

Sea salt and lime grilled fish tacos

Chapter 1 – Introduction to leptin and leptin resistance

If you're reading this you may be wondering "just what is leptin?"

Leptin is a hormone in your body that is essential in the regulation of your appetite and metabolism. Leptin production levels in your body, if not functioning correctly, can lead to quite a few problems including obesity and the feeling of feeling hungry all the time.

Leptin reacts with the cell receptors in your brain's hypothalamus gland to signal to the body when you've had enough to eat and feel full.

Leptin is produced mostly in your body's fat cells but it can also be made in much smaller amounts by the ovaries, pituitary gland, the liver, and even your bone marrow.

What causes leptin resistance isn't fully understood but there are theories as to what causes it.

The first theory is that leptin in the blood is not reaching the right targets to control a person's appetite.

The second theory is that the receptors that leptin binds itself to stop functioning properly and causes the cells to fail to respond the hormone. Though it can be difficult to work with leptin resistance there are things out there that can help you including, but not limited to diet and exercise. Working with leptin resistance will be a life style change but it does not have to be a difficult one.

Chapter 2 – Leptin resistance diet (what to eat what to reduce)

When dealing with leptin resistance it is important to eat healthy and balanced meals. Your doctor may prescribe a supplement for you to take to help you.

During this time you will want to eat healthy foods and having as much of a balanced meal plan as possible.

Your doctor will want to start you out on five rules that you will need to follow.

1. Never eat after dinner. This may be a hard rule to start enforcing but it will

become habit after time. Try finish eating a balanced dinner at least three hours before bed.

2. Eat three meals a day. Do your best to allow five to six hours between meals. Unless medically necessary avoid snaking!

3. Don't eat large meals. Finish your meal when you are feeling slightly less than feeling full.

4. Eat a high protein breakfast. The protein will help you avoid that crash later.

5. Reduce your carb intake. Again, this one can be hard at first but it will become easier as you work at it.

During this time you will want to avoid

- Sugar

- Fructose

- Processed foods

It is recommended that you eat a healthy diet with whole foods. If possible try replacing grain carbs with no to low sugar.

Lean protein is healthy for you so it is a good idea to eat a low to moderate amount of lean proteins each day.

You will also want to be eating healthy fats to help you with your diet. Omega-3 fats and krill oil are also good for you during this time. Krill oil can often be found in tablet form in the vitamin isle.

Superfoods are highly recommended and can help balance your leptin levels.

These superfoods include but are not limited to

- Basil

- Flaxseeds

- Romaine lettuce

- Some blueberry juices

- Some vegetable juices

- Carrots

- Green teas

- Broccoli

- Apples

- Almonds

- Walnuts

- Nonfat yogurt

Many of these items can be found at your local grocery store. Your doctor may send you to a nutritionist to help you find certain foods that can help you.

Chapter 3 – Breakfast recipes

Despite being on a specific diet to help you control and lose weight it does not mean that you will have to deprive yourself of healthy and tasty food. There are many great types of foods available to you!

They say breakfast is the most important meal of the day so why not start out with these great tasting meals?

Raspberry vanilla oatmeal

This is an easy to make oatmeal that you make the night before. It's loaded with the good stuff that you need and will help keep you going through the day.

Ingredients

- Three fourth cup of uncooked oats

- One half cup of almond milk

- One tablespoon of date paste

- One half teaspoon of vanilla extract

- Pinch of salt

- Water

Instructions

Place all the ingredients save for the raspberries in a bowl and mix well. Cover and place in your refrigerator overnight.

When you are ready for the oatmeal sprinkle sliced almonds and raspberries over it and serve cold.

Tomato borscht

Here's something tasty that will provide you with almost everything you need for the day!

Ingredients

- Two tablespoons of olive oil

- One small onion, chopped

- One clove of garlic, chopped

- Eight ounces of raw beetroot, peeled and grated

- One teaspoon of ground toasted cumin seeds

- One fourth teaspoon of ground cinnamon

- Eight ounces of ripe fresh tomatoes, chopped

- Eight ounces of tomato juice

- One tablespoon of sun dried tomatoes, chopped

- One pint of vegetable stock

- One tablespoon of light soy sauce

- Salt

- Ground black pepper

- Toasted cumin seeds

- Soured cream

Instructions

Heat up a large pan and cook the olive oil, onions, and garlic.

After five minutes have passed add the beetroot and cook until brown. This should take about five minutes.

Once five minutes have passed add all the other ingredients except for the soy sauce. Allow this mixture to cook for fifteen minutes before adding the soy sauce.

This can be served chilled or warm depending on your preferences.

Kale salad

This tasty salad is savory, sweet, and spicy. It may just be what you're looking for!

Ingredients

- One bunch of organic kale

- One half cup of cooked chickpeas

- One third of a small sweet onion, thinly sliced

- One third cup of raisins

- One third cup of organic sesame tahini

- One half cup of lemon juice

- Pinch of cayenne or paprika

- One teaspoon of salt

Instructions

In a large bowl mix everything except for the sesame tahini, lemon juice, cayenne, and salt. In a separate bowl combine the sesame tahini, lemon juice, cayenne, and salt as this will become your dressing.

Place your salad in a bowl and pour your dressing over it and enjoy.

Roasted beet and goat cheese salad

If you wish to try something different for breakfast this can be a great place to start. Even if you don't have the time in the morning you can make this the night before and save it.

Ingredients

- Four medium sized beets

- Two cups organic baby arugula (or spinach)

- Three ounces goat cheese

- One half small red onion, thinly sliced

- One half cup pinenuts (optional)

- One fourth cup olive oil

Dressing

- One fourth cup extra virgin olive oil

- Two tablespoons white balsamic vinegar (or lemon juice)

- One tablespoon dried oregano

- Salt

- Pepper

Instructions

Preheat your oven to 375 degrees F. Place the beets in a shallow baking dish and pour just over half the olive oil in it. Roll the beats in it to coat and cover.

Bake until tender. This should take about ninety minutes. Remove from the oven to cool. Once cool skin the beats and cut them into one inch pieces.

Mix all the dressing ingredients together and set aside.

When ready to eat assemble the salad by placing the greens on a salad plate. Arrange the beat slices and onion slices on top.

Drizzle the dressing on top but just enough on it to lightly coat everything.

Crumble the goat cheese and use it as the garnish.

Chapter 4 – Lunch Recipes

Lunch is also an important meal of the day but it does not mean that you have to be deprived. Try these four healthy and tasty lunch meals anytime!

Chicken Chili

If you enjoy chicken chili here is a healthy and tasty way to enjoy it! If you wish for extra spiciness you can add red pepper flakes or diced green chilies. After cooking the chicken chili you can also top it with cilantro.

Ingredients

- One tablespoon of olive oil

- One pound organic chicken breast, cubed

- One cup of onions, diced

- One fifteen ounce jar of stewed tomatoes

- One fifteen ounce can of organic white beans

- One fifteen ounce can of organic black beans

- Two cloves of garlic, minced

- One fresh jalapeno, seeded and diced

- Two tablespoon of chili powder

- One half teaspoon dried oregano

- One fourth teaspoon ground cumin

- Salt

- Pepper

Instructions

Coat your skillet with the olive oil. Add the chicken and onions and brown them over a low-medium heat until cooked through.

Add the other ingredients and cook on a low heat for approximately fifteen to twenty minutes. Once cooked pour into bowls and enjoy.

Crab salad

Who doesn't enjoy a good salad? This salad is also loaded with avocado, apples, and green beans so you won't be missing out on anything.

Ingredients

- One and one half cups green beans, trimmed at both ends, cut into one half inch pieces

- Two tablespoons coarse sea salt

- One cup Greek style yogurt

- One tablespoon Dijon mustard

- One fourth teaspoon fine sea salt

- Four tablespoons minced fresh chives

- One Granny Smith apple, peeled and cubed

- One ripe avocado, peeled and cubed

- One cup (eight ounces) cooked lump crabmeat

Instructions

Fill a large pot that is fitted with a colander with water. Place over a high heat and bring to a roaring boil. Add the green beans and coarse sea salt to the colander and cook until tender. This should take three to four minutes.

Remove the colander from the pot and rinse the beans with cold water, drain, and pat dry with a clean paper towel.

In a large bowl whisk the yogurt, mustard, and fine sea salt. Add the green beans, chives, apple, avocado, and crab meat. Toss well and enjoy.

Sea salt and lime grilled fish tacos

Here's another healthy and tasty recipe for you to try! Why spend big money at a restaurant when you can make your own great tasting tacos for a fraction of the price?

Ingredients

- One pound (one inch thick) halibut fish fillets

- One fourth cup lime juice

- One fourth cup chopped fresh cilantro

- One fourth cup olive oil

- One fourth cup prepared salsa verde or pico de gallo

- One jalepeno, diced (optional)

- One fourth cup organic mayonnaise

- One teaspoon sea salt, divided

- One cup shredded green cabbage

- One cup shredded red cabbage

- Sixteen avocado slices (about two small avocados)

- Eight corn (or whole wheat flour) tortillas

- Two limes, cut in half

Instructions

Preheat your grill to a medium-high heat.

In a large plastic bag with a zip closure combine the lime juice, cilantro, oil, and halibut. Marinade in the refrigerator for twenty minutes.

For the creamy salsa verde combine the salsa, jalepeno and mayonnaise in a blender. Puree until smooth.

Remove the fish from the marinade and season with one half teaspoon sea salt and place on the hot grill. Grill the fish for six minutes on each side and remove. Let sit for several minutes and then flake the fish with a fork.

Place the lime halves on the grill, flesh side down, along with the tortillas for one minutes or until the limes are grill marked and one side of the tortillas are toasted. Remove and bend the tortillas toasted side out into a taco like shape.

Fill each tortilla with one fourth cup slaw and two slices of avocado. Divide the fish evenly among the tacos and drizzle each with one tablespoon sauce. Sprinkle the remaining sea salt and serve with a grilled lime half.

Fresh caprese quinoa salad

Here's an easy to make, unique, and tasty salad to try!

Ingredients

- One half cup organic quinoa

- Eight ounces fresh mozzarella

- One carton grape tomatoes, halved

- Fresh basil, chopped

- Two tablespoons extra virgin olive oil

- Kosher salt

- Pepper

Instructions

In a medium sized pan add one cup filtered water and bring to a boil. Add one half cup quinoa. Reduce the heat and simmer on low until all of the water is absorbed. This should take about fifteen minutes.

Cool the cooked quinoa in your refrigerator for at least one hour.

Slice the grape tomatoes in half the long way.
Cut the ball of mozzarella cheese into bite sized
pieces and mix together.
Toss in the chopped basil and cooked quinoa.
Drizzle on the olive oil and season with a little
salt and pepper.
This salad can be served cool or at room
temperature.

Chapter 5 – Dinner Recipes

A healthy dinner will go a long way in helping you control your weight and leptin. Below are four great tasting and easy to make recipes!

Seared salmon with roasted asparagus

If you enjoy salmon this is an excellent recipe to try.

Ingredients

- One and one fourth pounds wild Alaskan salmon fillet

- One tablespoon chopped fresh rosemary (or one teaspoon dried)

- One teaspoon salt

- One one and a half pounds fresh organic asparagus

- One one and a half tablespoons extra-virgin olive oil

- One small organic onion, diced

- Two tablespoons pine nuts

- One cup filtered water

- One half cup brown rice

Instructions

While your oven is heating up season the salmon half of the rosemary and one half teaspoon salt for twenty minutes and up to one hour before cooking. Let the salmon sit while you prepare the other food.

Preheat your oven to 425 degrees F.

Prepare the brown rice by adding one cup filtered water to a pot and bring it to a boil. Add one half cup of the brown rice and turn the heat down to low. Cover the pot and let it cook for thirty five to forty minutes.

Snap off the bottoms of the asparagus ends. Season the asparagus with one half teaspoon salt and some oil. Toss these to combine. Place the asparagus on a sheet and cook it for eight to ten minutes.

Heat one tablespoon oil in a large and wide sauce pan over medium heat. Add the diced onion and cook while stirring occasionally until translucent. This should take three to four minutes.

Add the pine nuts and remaining rosemary. Cook while stirring until the pine nuts are beginning to brown. This should take an additional three to five minutes.

Heat the last of the remaining oil in a large skillet over medium-high heat. Add the salmon with the skinned side up and cook until a golden brown. Turn the salmon over and remove the pan from the heat and let stand until just cooked through. This should take three to five minutes. When ready to serve layer the food so that the brown rice is on the bottom, the salmon in the middle, and the nuts and any remaining liquid on top.

Shrimp with garlic sauce

If you enjoy shrimp this is an easy recipe to make that you and others are sure to enjoy!

Ingredients

- One and one half pounds uncooked large wild shrimp

- Three tablespoons Tamari sauce

- Two tablespoons chili sauce

- Two teaspoons sesame oil

- Two teaspoons rice wine

- Two tablespoons olive oil

- Three gloves garlic minced

- One scallion, thinly sliced

- Black pepper (to taste)

Instructions

Peel the shrimp but leave the tail segments intact. After the shrimp are peeled devein them. In a small bowl mix the Tamari sauce, chili sauce, sesame oil, and rice wine. Mix well and set aside.

In a large pan heat the olive oil over medium-high heat. Stir fry the garlic until it is fragrant. This should take thirty seconds.

Add the shrimp and cook until both sides are pink. This should take about two minutes on each side.

Add the sauce mixture and stir until the shrimp are fully coated.

Season with black pepper.

Remove the pan from the heat and garnish with chopped scallions.

Serve with brown rice and/or vegetables.

Chicken kabobs

Kabobs can be fun to make and these chicken kabobs are as good for you as they are tasty.

Ingredients

- Three tablespoons Tamari

- One tablespoon extra-virgin olive oil

- Juice from one lime

- One teaspoon garlic, minced

- Four skinless, boneless chicken breast halves

- Cilantro (to taste)

Instructions

In a small bowl combine and mix the Tamari sauce, extra virgin olive oil, a handful of chopped cilantro, lime juice, and garlic. Set aside.

Cut the chicken into large chunks and skewer them onto bamboo sticks that have been soaked in water for five minutes. Allow to marinate for at least thirty minutes.

Grill the kabobs on medium high heat for six to eight minutes on each side or until the juices are clear.

Serve with a fresh salad or steamed vegetables.

Steak burritos

Steak burritos for a great alternative for dinner on occasion. These easy to make and tasty burritos should become a favorite in no time!

Ingredients

Marinade:

- Two jalapenos, seeded and diced

- One fourth cup cumin seeds, toasted

- Three fourth cup olive oil

- One bunch cilantro (stems and leaves)

- One teaspoon salt

- One tablespoon black pepper

- One clove garlic, crushed

- One half cup lime juice

Rice, steak, burrito:

- One half cup prepared fresh salsa

- One half cup water

- One fourth cup uncooked long grain brown rice

- One fifteen ounce can black beans

- Twelve ounces grass-fed strip steak, trimmed and thinly sliced crosswise

- One tablespoon olive oil

- Four eight inch whole-wheat or brown rice tortillas

- One half cup shredded sharp cheddar cheese

- One fourth cup fresh guacamole (or avocado slices)

- Two tablespoons coarsely chopped fresh cilantro

Instructions

Marinade

Place all the marinade ingredients in a blender and blend until smooth. Pour the marinade blend over the beef slices. Cover and place in the refrigerator overnight.

Cook the rice via your preferred method or by the directions. When there are ten minutes left in the cooking time add the salsa and water to the rice and simmer for five minutes.

Stir in the beans and simmer uncooked until the rice is tender and most of the liquid has been absorbed. This should take about five minutes.

While that cooks heat the oil in a large skillet over medium-high heat. Add the steak slices and cook while stirring occasionally until the meat is browned and cooked through. This should take three to five minutes.

When you are ready to prepare the burrito divide the steak among the tortillas and top with equal amounts of cheese, guacamole, cilantro, and the rice mixture.

Roll each tortilla into a burrito and enjoy.

Chapter 6 – Dessert Recipes

I couldn't leave you hanging and forget all about tasty deserts! Many of these are easy to make and are quite tasty.

Chocolate smoothie

If you like chocolate here's a great recipe to try! It's so simple you may wonder why you haven't thought of it first!

Ingredients

- One scoop of daily protein chocolate

- One cup of 2% milk

- One fourth teaspoon of cayenne pepper

- One half teaspoon of cinnamon

- One tablespoon of honey

- Four ice cubes

Instructions

Place all of the ingredients inside a blender and puree until smooth or until it reaches your desired consistency.

Cucumber mint cooler

If chocolate isn't your thing here's another great smoothie to try!

Ingredients

- One scoop of unflavored dairy protein

- One cup of chopped cucumbers

- One fourth cup chopped mint

- One cup water

- Four ice cubes

- One teaspoon honey

Instructions

Place all of the ingredients inside a blender and puree until smooth or until it reaches your desired consistency.

Yogurt parfait

Why spend the money buying a yogurt parfait when you can make your own for a fraction of the cost? Not only will it be healthy for you you'll know exactly what's going into it!

Ingredients

- One cup organic plain yogurt (make sure it is antibiotics and hormone free)

- One fourth cup organic raw granola (it should have no sweetener)

- One fourth cup organic Goji berries, dried

- Organic honey (optional and for more sweetness if desired)

Instructions

In a medium sized bowl add the granola, goji berries, yogurt, and honey and stir to mix well. Carefully scoop the mixture into serving dishes and top with the remaining granola and goji berries.

Chocolate chip cookies

These chocolate cookies are nut, grain, and dairy free but are full of flavor!

Ingredients

- Seven tablespoons palm shortening

- One third cup plus two tablespoons coconut sugar

- One tablespoon raw honey

- One large egg

- One third cup coconut flour

- One third cup tapioca flour

- One third cup arrowroot flour

- One half teaspoon Celtic sea salt

- One teaspoon baking soda

- Three fourth teaspoon unflavored, grass-fed gelatin

- One cup Enjoy Life chocolate chips or chunks

Instructions

Preheat your oven to 350 degrees F and adjust the rack into the middle position.

Inside the bowl for a mixer add the palm shortening, sugar, and honey. Beat on medium-high for two minutes.

Scrape the sides of the bowl and add in the egg.

In a separate large bowl sift the coconut flour, tapioca flour, arrowroot flour, sea salt, baking soda, and gelatin.

With the mixer on low slowly add in the dry mixture into the wet mixture.

Stir in the chocolate chips.

Using a spoon scoop and make dough balls onto a baking sheet lined with unbleached parchment paper.

Bake for eleven minutes and enjoy.

Conclusion on the Leptin Diet

Thank you again for downloading this book! I really hope you've enjoyed reading all about the leptin diet and its proven strategies on how to tackle it effectively.

Make sure you also check out my other health books on adrenal fatigue and anti-inflammatory diet which are always full of fresh new ideas to help you benefits from this healthy way of life.

The next step is to take action on what you have learned today. I'm sure with the right practice and listening to my directions step by step of the way you will create a better happy, healthy and more vibrant lifestyle for yourself.

Finally, if you enjoyed this book, then I'd like to ask you for a favor, would you be kind enough to leave a review for this book on Amazon? It'd be greatly appreciated!

Bon Apetite,

Kathy Hunt

Free Preview of my "Adrenal Fatigue Book"

Adrenal Fatigue

Reset Your Adrenal Health Naturally

By Kathy Hunt

Chapter 1 – What is adrenal fatigue?

Adrenal fatigue is not caused by solely one particular thing in the body and is also not always widely accepted by the medical community.

Adrenal fatigue is a collection of signs and symptoms that result when your adrenal glands function below the necessary level for health and survival.

This can be brought on by intense and/or prolonged stress, acute or chronic infections, influenza, bronchitis, and pneumonia. While these are common signs they are not the only ones that can cause it.

A person with adrenal fatigue can look and act perfectly normal and healthy which may lead to surprise when someone learns that person is actually ill.

Many people with adrenal fatigue may feel unwell, tired, or feeling off kilter emotions wise. Many people who are experiencing this condition will use caffeine and other stimulants to keep themselves going through the day.

Adrenal fatigue is caused when your adrenal glands cannot meet the demands of stress you may be feeling. Your adrenal glands are important in your body's response to every type of stress be it physical, emotional, and/or psychological.

The adrenal glands help with hormones that regulate your body's energy production, storage, immune function, heart rate, muscle tone, and other process that help you cope with the stress you are feeling. If the response from the adrenal glands is inadequate to what you need it can cause adrenal fatigue.

Adrenal fatigue can wreak great havoc in your life. This can be mild to severe where the adrenal glands are in such bad shape that a person may have difficulty getting out of bed for more than a few hours per day.

Because of this the other organs inside the body are negatively affected. Because the adrenal glands are so badly affected the rest of your body goes into over drive to compensation and make up for the adrenal glands. This may work for a short time but soon your body becomes more fatigued and negatively affected.

Adrenal fatigue has also been known by many other names in history. These names include non-Addison's hypoadrenia, sub-clinical hypoadrenia, neurasthenia, adrenal neurasthenia, adrenal apathy and adrenal fatigue.

Though not widely recognized in medicine adrenal fatigue affects millions of people worldwide. Anyone can fall victim to adrenal fatigue as this condition does not know age, race, or gender. Despite how frightening this may sound there **is** help available to you!

Chapter 2 – Symptoms and signs of adrenal fatigue

The symptoms of adrenal fatigue can vary from person to person and even from gender to gender.

These symptoms can include but are not limited to

- Hollow cheeks

- Vertical lines in the finger nails

- Unexplained back and/or knee pain

- Fatigue

- Body aches

- Unexplained weight loss

- Low blood pressure

- Lightheadedness

- Loss of body hair. These bald patches are most noticed on the legs and arms.

- Hyperpigmentation (skin discoloration)

- Non-refreshing sleep even if you're getting enough hours of sleep

- Feeling confused or like you're in a frequent "brain fog"

- Craving salty and/or sweet foods

- Consistent low blood pressure

- Extreme sensitivity to cold

- Weakened immune system

- Menopause problems

- Decreased sex drive

- Increased allergies or sudden new allergies develop

- Inability to handle stressful situations

- Depression

- Light sensitivity

Adrenal Fatigue Soup

This is a great soup as it helps balance your body.

Ingredients

- Sixteen ounces green beans

- One cup chopped celery

- One zucchini, sliced

- One medium onion, chopped

- One cup tomato juice

- One cup spring water

- Two tablespoons raw honey

- One teaspoon paprika

- One cup chicken broth

Instructions

Combine all the ingredients into a large soup pot and let simmer for one hour or until the vegetables are tender.

Season with pepper to taste.

Adrenal Support Smoothie

This is a tasty and healthy smoothie you can work into your diet. It is not meant to replace a meal but may be used in addition to.

Ingredients

- One cup green tea, chilled or room temp

- One half medium avocado

- One half cup fresh or frozen blueberries

- One half tablespoon maca

- One half teaspoon ginger spice or fresh ginger, grated

- Dash of Celtic sea salt

- One half tablespoon raw honey to sweeten

Optional additional ingredients

- One teaspoon ashwaganda powder

- One teaspoon Siberian ginseng

- One cup spinach or kale

- Cacao

- Goji berries

- Coconut oil

- Bee pollen

- Spirulina

Instructions

Place all the ingredients inside a blender and blend well for thirty to forty five seconds or until your desired consistency is reached.

The information herein is offered for informational purposes solely, and is universal as so. The presentation of the information is without contract or any type of guarantee assurance.

The trademarks that are used are without any consent, and the publication of the trademark is without permission or backing by the trademark owner. All trademarks and brands within this book are for clarifying purposes only and are the owned by the owners themselves, not affiliated with this document.

www.ingramcontent.com/pod-product-compliance
Lightning Source LLC
Chambersburg PA
CBHW072025290526
45787CB00015B/2203